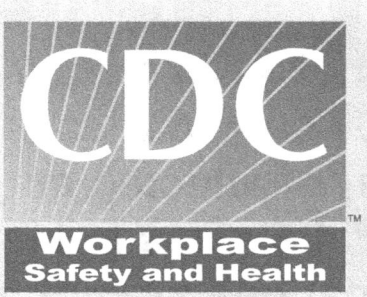

I0426398

Evaluation of 1-Bromopropane Use in Four New Jersey Commercial Dry Cleaning Facilities

Judith Eisenberg, MD, MS
Jessica Ramsey, MS

Health Hazard Evaluation Report
HETA 2008-0175-3111
New Jersey Department of Health and Senior Services
July 2010

Department of Health and Human Services
Centers for Disease Control and Prevention

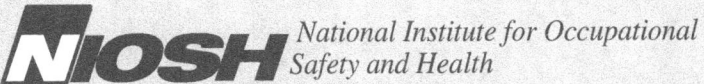

National Institute for Occupational Safety and Health

The employer shall post a copy of this report for a period of 30 calendar days at or near the workplace(s) of affected employees. The employer shall take steps to insure that the posted determinations are not altered, defaced, or covered by other material during such period. [37 FR 23640, November 7, 1972, as amended at 45 FR 2653, January 14, 1980].

CONTENTS

ABBREVIATIONS

1-BP	1-bromopropane
ACGIH®	American Conference of Governmental Industrial Hygienists
cc/min	Cubic centimeters per minute
CDC	Centers for Disease Control and Prevention
cfm	Cubic feet per minute
CFR	Code of Federal Regulations
CT	Computed tomography
ED	Emergency department
ft^2	square feet
IARC	International Agency for Research on Cancer
LEV	Local exhaust ventilation
LOD	Limit of detection
LOQ	Limit of quantification
mcg/mL	Micrograms per milliliter
meq/L	Milliequivalents per liter
mg/L	Milligrams per liter
μg/sample	Micrograms per sample
MMWR	Morbidity and Mortality Weekly Report
NAICS	North American Industry Classification System
NIOSH	National Institute for Occupational Safety and Health
NJ DEP	New Jersey Department of Environmental Protection
NJ DHSS	New Jersey Department of Health and Senior Services
OEL	Occupational exposure limit
OSHA	Occupational Safety and Health Administration
PBZ	Personal breathing zone
PEL	Permissible exposure limit
perc	Perchloroethylene
PPE	Personal protective equipment
ppm	Parts per million
REL	Recommended exposure limit
STEL	Short term exposure limit
TLV®	Threshold limit value
TWA	Time-weighted average
U.S. EPA	United States Environmental Protection Agency
WEEL	Workplace environmental exposure limit

HIGHLIGHTS OF THE NIOSH HEALTH HAZARD EVALUATION

> The National Institute for Occupational Safety and Health (NIOSH) received a technical assistance request from the New Jersey Department of Health and Senior Services. The request concerned a report of health effects in an operator using 1-bromopropane (1-BP) at a dry cleaning facility.

What NIOSH Did

- In August 2008, we visited four dry cleaning facilities that had converted their systems from perchloroethylene (perc) to 1-BP.

- We interviewed owners, operators, and an employee about their work and any symptoms they thought were work related. We later reviewed medical records.

- We collected air samples for 1-BP at the same facilities in November 2008.

What NIOSH Found

- An operator reported lightheadedness when cooking 1-BP. This is a symptom that can occur with general solvent use.

- No cases of peripheral neuropathy were found among owners, operators, or employees.

- Work practices, how conversions were done, and the amount of 1-BP used varied widely.

- Operators who converted machines on their own or who cooked 1-BP were exposed to high concentrations of 1-BP in the air.

- Respirators, gloves, and eye protection were not being used. Respirators were not equipped with the correct cartridges for 1-BP.

What Owners Can Do

- Use a qualified technician to convert the machines from perc to 1-BP.

- Follow the manufacturer's guidelines for safe product use. This includes the use of ventilation, specific temperatures, and appropriate system settings.

- Use general building ventilation to reduce 1-BP concentrations in the air.

- Use local exhaust ventilation or open the doors to outside when loading or unloading machines, pouring solvent, and maintaining equipment.

What Operators Can Do

- Do not cook 1-BP or cut the drying periods short as this may increase 1-BP exposures to operators.

- Wear eye protection, gloves, and a respirator when handling 1-BP.

- If personal air monitoring indicates the above steps are not effective at reducing exposures below applicable occupational exposure limits, then respiratory protection should be used. Employees should be fit tested and trained how to use and store respirators properly.

What Owners, Operators, and Employees Can Do

- If you become lightheaded, short of breath, or nauseated, or develop a headache when handling 1-BP, stop immediately and go outside. If symptoms do not resolve within minutes or if you develop muscle weakness or sensory problems, seek care at the nearest emergency department. Tell the healthcare provider about your workplace exposure to 1-BP.

SUMMARY

We found no cases of peripheral neuropathy among dry cleaners who had switched from perc to 1-BP. 1-BP levels that exceeded the ACGIH TLV-TWA of 10 ppm were found. We recommend that dry cleaning facilities using 1-BP as a perc alternative use a qualified technician to convert the machines.

On May 2, 2008, NIOSH received a technical assistance request from the NJ DHSS regarding potential health effects of 1-BP in drycleaners. This solvent can be used in the same machine as perc after a conversion process. One New Jersey dry cleaner owner required medical evaluation after becoming symptomatic while doing the 1-BP conversion himself. Initial reports indicated the possibility of peripheral neuropathy. Because 1-BP has been documented in the medical literature to cause peripheral neuropathy, NIOSH was asked to evaluate possible exposures and health effects among dry cleaner operators who used 1-BP.

In August 2008, we visited four of eight facilities in New Jersey that had been approved to use 1-BP in dry cleaning operations. We interviewed owners, operators, and an employee about the conversion process, work practices, and adverse health effects they associated with 1-BP use. PBZ and area air sampling was performed during normal operation of the 1-BP system during our second site visit in November 2008.

Six interviews were conducted with owners, operators, and employees. One person reported transient lightheadedness, which is consistent with general solvent exposure. The owner who sought prior medical care for symptoms that occurred while handling 1-BP had no residual neurological deficits at the time of our visit. Review of this individual's medical records did not reveal neurological abnormalities at an ED visit when symptoms first developed, and serum bromide levels obtained during that ED visit were well under levels associated with adverse health effects.

Full-shift sampling for 1-BP conducted at one of the facilities resulted in PBZ air concentrations of 40 ppm for the operator and 17 ppm for the cashier. PBZ concentrations ranging from 1.5 to 160 ppm were found in partial shift samples taken at the other three facilities. These results confirmed the release of 1-BP into the environment at all four locations, indicating a potential hazard to employees.

We recommend that dry cleaner operators using 1-BP as a perc alternative use a qualified technician to convert the machines. Operators should not cook the solvent nor cut drying periods short, as doing so may increase exposure to 1-BP. Until 1-BP exposures can be consistently documented to be below the OEL, respirators are recommended. Use of respirators should occur within the setting of a comprehensive respiratory protection program. General ventilation should always be used to dilute 1-BP concentrations in the air.

Symptoms such as lightheadedness, headache, and nausea are consistent with solvent exposure. If employees notice these symptoms they should leave the area. Employees should not resume work until the source of the exposure has been indentified and corrected. If symptoms do not resolve shortly after leaving the work area, employees should seek immediate medical attention and inform their healthcare provider of their potential exposure to 1-BP.

Keywords: NAICS 812320 (Dry Cleaning and Laundry Services (except Coin-Operated)), dry cleaning, 1-bromopropane, n-propyl bromide, solvent, neuropathy

On May 2, 2008, NIOSH received a request for technical assistance from the NJ DHSS regarding potential health effects from exposure to 1-BP (1-bromopropane), also known as n-propyl bromide, and marketed under the trade names of Dry-Solv™ and Fabri-Solv™. The request was prompted by a suspected case of peripheral neuropathy in an owner of a dry cleaning establishment who had handled a large amount of 1-BP while converting a machine to 1-BP operations. The dry cleaning businesses we visited are small establishments. The owner is the individual responsible for making business decisions. Operators are those personnel who refill the machines with 1-BP and who load and unload clothes from the machine. Often the owner is also an operator. Employees, such as cashiers and press machine operators work in the facility but do not work with the dry-cleaning machine containing 1-BP.

Background

Perc has been the solvent of choice in commercial dry cleaning for more than 50 years. In December 2007, the administrator of New Jersey's Bureau of Air Compliance and Enforcement in the NJ DEP estimated that 1500 of the 1700 dry cleaning facilities in the state utilized perc systems [McAneny 2007].

Although the IARC recognizes perc as a probable human carcinogen, its use has only recently been restricted in the United States because of its ozone depletion properties and environmental pollution contributions. Perc was noted to be one of the top ten air contaminants in New Jersey and has also been identified as a source of soil and water pollution [NJ DEP 2010a]. The U.S. EPA will ban the use of perc in coresidential dry cleaning facilities as of December 20, 2020 [40 CFR 63.323(5) (i)]. In 2007, California became the first state to ban perc use in dry cleaning ahead of the federal ban, and other states, such as North Carolina, New York, and Massachusetts, are contemplating similar actions. More recently, the NJ DEP has encouraged owners to replace their perc machines with hydrocarbon dry cleaning systems or professional wet cleaning systems [NJ DEP 2010b].

Several perc alternatives are available to dry cleaning owners, including 1-BP, aliphatic hydrocarbons (DF-2000), silicone-based cleaner (GreenEarth®), carbon dioxide, and wet cleaning methods. However, 1-BP is the only perc alternative that can be used in the original perc machines with alterations. The cost of converting an existing perc machine to use 1-BP is approximately $4,000, compared to approximately $50,000 to buy a new machine that uses aliphatic hydrocarbon or silicone-based cleaners. A 2007 nationwide industry survey revealed that of those owners who were considering replacing their perc systems, 24% would choose to convert to 1-BP [American Drycleaner 2007]. The NJ DEP has instituted a reimbursement program offering grants to owners to help offset the costs of switching to nonperc systems [NJ DEP 2010b].

INTRODUCTION
(CONTINUED)

Anticipated increased use of 1-BP as a perc alternative suggests the need for a better understanding of the exposures of dry cleaner operators and potential adverse health effects. High 1-BP exposures in electronics degreasing and foam cushion manufacturing have resulted in cases of peripheral neuropathy in employees [NIOSH 2001; NIOSH 2002; NIOSH 2003]. In some cases, these neurologic deficits were permanent. In February 2008, the NJ DHSS was made aware of one dry cleaning owner believed to have developed symptoms consistent with peripheral neuropathy during an exposure to 1-BP, which prompted its request to NIOSH for technical assistance. At the time of the request, eight dry cleaning facilities in the state were licensed to use 1-BP; four of these facilities consented to participate in the NIOSH evaluation.

ASSESSMENT

On August 26–28, 2008, we made initial site visits to the four dry cleaning facilities, and interviewed the owners, operators, and an employee about the conversion process from perc to 1-BP, work practices involving 1-BP, and health effects related to 1-BP. Medical records release forms were completed by the owner who was evaluated for possible 1-BP related symptoms, and these records were reviewed.

On November 18–20, 2008, we returned to the facilities to collect PBZ and area air samples for 1-BP. We collected PBZ air samples on the operators who ran the machines and the cashiers at the front of the store who received and distributed items. The employees wore sampling devices with the sample media placed in their breathing zones. Area samples were collected in various places around the shops, including behind the machines to quantify exposures from any leaks. Air samples were only collected during times when the dry cleaning equipment was operating because the owners requested we stop monitoring when they stopped using the 1-BP machines. We collected air samples using NIOSH Method 1025 for 1-BP [NIOSH 2009]. In this method, air is drawn through a standard charcoal tube (SKC Anasorb® CSC Lot 4936) using a calibrated personal sampling pump at a nominal flow rate of 50 cc/min. After sampling, the charcoal tubes were capped and shipped refrigerated to the analytical laboratory. Samples were analyzed for 1-BP using gas chromatography with flame ionization detection. The 1-BP LOD was 1 µg/sample, and the LOQ was 4 µg/sample. The OELs and potential health effects for 1-BP are discussed in Appendix A.

RESULTS

Health Concerns

A published report of the owner exposed to 1-BP stated that he experienced symptoms of headaches, fatigue, visual disturbances, tremors, and "muscle twitching" [CDC 2008]. During our interview with this owner regarding the incident, he recalled a slightly different set of symptoms including headache, shortness of breath, fatigue, and chest tightness while converting his machine to 1-BP from perc. He contacted the local poison control center and was advised to report to the nearest ED for evaluation. Review of his ED medical records showed that the physical examination, chest x-ray, and head CT were normal. The only abnormality on the standard blood tests was an elevated serum chloride level of 110 meq/L (reference range: 96–106 meq/L). A serum bromide level was ordered during his ED visit, but the laboratory that analyzed the sample did not have this result available until 4 days after the visit. As per the reporting laboratory, bromide toxicity is expected with serum levels greater than or equal to 1250 mcg/mL, which is much higher than the 144 mcg/mL level reported for this owner [Quest Diagnostics Incorporated, Chantilly, Virginia]. This owner reported no persistent neurological deficits and developed no signs or symptoms that would indicate a need for an evaluation by a neurologist.

Another owner reported often feeling lightheaded and "buzzed" while handling 1-BP particularly when "cooking" the solvent (boiling the solvent to remove impunties). These symptoms resolved minutes after he went outside. None of those interviewed reported persistent weakness, sensation deficits, or balance disturbances.

Environmental Sampling

PBZ air sampling results for 1-BP are included in Table 1.

Table 1. Personal breathing zone air concentrations of 1-BP at four dry cleaning facilities

Job Title	# of Loads	Cooking	Sampling Time (minutes)	Concentration (ppm)	Full Shift TWA (ppm)
Operator – Facility 1			07:43 – 11:43 (241)	56	40
			11:45 – 15:44 (240)	23	
	10	Yes			
Cashier – Facility 1			07:44 – 11:47 (243)	24	17
			11:47 – 15:52 (245)	10	
Operator – Facility 2			08:35 – 12:04 (209)	7.2	N/A*
	3	No			
Cashier – Facility 2			08:37 – 12:09 (212)	1.5	N/A
Operator – Facility 3	1	No	07:10 – 09:52 (163)	11	N/A
Operator – Facility 4			11:43 – 15:43 (241)	160	N/A
	1	Yes			
Cashier – Facility 4			11:41 – 15:45 (246)	2.4	N/A

*N/A = not applicable

Facility 1 was using a Multimatic 35-pound machine (Multimatic, Northvale, New Jersey). The machine had been converted from perc to 1-BP by the owner. During sampling, 10 loads of dry cleaning were run. No solvent was added to the machine during the sampling period. Although most modern machines can run multiple loads through an automated software program, the operator at this facility manually ran each load and cooked after every load. Full-shift TWA exposures were calculated for the owner/operator (40 ppm) and cashier (17 ppm). Other employees were using press machines next to the dry cleaning machine while the cashier moved around the shop retrieving finished items and handling customer transactions. Area air samples were collected behind (103 ppm in the morning and 48 ppm in the afternoon) and in front (66 ppm in the morning and 36 ppm in the afternoon) of the dry cleaning machine for approximately 8 hours. In the morning, at the beginning of the sampling period, the building's ventilation system was off, the doors were closed, and the front windows were open. In the afternoon, the back door was open, and the ventilation system was on to improve dilution and air mixing.

Facility 2 was using a VIC 35-pound machine (Dalex, Concord, Ontario). The machine had been converted by Enviro Tech International, the company that provided this dry cleaner with the 1-BP material. During sampling, three loads of dry cleaning were run. No solvent was added to the machine during the sampling period, and no cooking was performed. An oscillating fan next to the door of the dry cleaning machine was on during the sampling period. The fan blew air towards the operator as he loaded and unloaded the machine. Other employees were using press machines next to the dry cleaning machine; after the operator had loaded and started the machine, he also used a press machine. The cashier in this facility mainly stayed in the front of the building taking clothing from customers, writing receipts, and handling payment transactions. Area air samples were collected behind (1.5 ppm) and in front (6.4 ppm) of the dry cleaning machine for the 3.5-hour sampling period while PBZ air sampling was performed.

Facility 3 used a Frimair 20–25-pound machine (Frimair, Turnersville, New Jersey). The machine had been converted to 1-BP use by Enviro Tech International. On the day of sampling, only one load of dry cleaning was run, and the operator had just started the load before we began sampling. The operator was the only employee on the premises, and he did the dry cleaning while also handling front counter duties, which included clothing intake, writing receipts for customers, and payment transactions. We collected an area air sample at the front counter that measured 8.6 ppm, similar to the operator's PBZ air concentration of 11 ppm. After the single run was completed, the operator explained that he would only perform counter duties for the remainder of the work day. Because he planned to do no more runs that day, the operator asked that we discontinue sampling at the end of the cycle. No solvent was added to the machine, and no cooking was performed during the sampling period.

Facility 4 was using a Frimair 30–35-pound machine (Frimair, Turnersville, New Jersey). The owner of the facility had converted the machine. During sampling, most of the operator's time was spent behind the machine, monitoring it while cooking the solvent. One load of dry cleaning was run at the end of the sampling period. Another employee performed the cashier duties in this facility; he also used a press machine next to the dry cleaning machine. Area air samples were collected behind (170 ppm) and in front (33 ppm) of the dry cleaning machine for the approximate 4-hour period that PBZ air sampling was performed. The front door of the facility was open, and a large building exhaust fan was on during the sampling period. The operator explained that he always ran the exhaust fan while he was cooking. Although he did cook solvent, none was added to the machine during the sampling period.

General Observations

None of the operators at the four locations used gloves or eye protection when handling or pouring the solvent. Two of the four operators had elastomeric half mask respirators; however, they did not have the correct organic vapor cartridges.

DISCUSSION

At the time of the request, eight dry cleaning facilities in the state of New Jersey were licensed by the NJ DEP to use 1-BP. We collected PBZ and area air samples at four of the eight locations that elected to participate in our evaluation. No two locations were performing the same amount or type of work, and work practices varied greatly, making comparisons difficult. The work volume at the facilities ranged from one to ten loads of dry cleaning over a workday, and some operators cooked the solvent, while others did not.

Because of initial reports that one owner had developed symptoms while using 1-BP, including some that were consistent with peripheral neuropathy, we were asked to focus on this health effect in our evaluation. Previous investigations have linked peripheral neuropathy to high-level 1-BP exposure in electronics degreasing [NIOSH 2001] and foam cushion manufacturing [NIOSH 2002; NIOSH 2003]. Case reports in the medical literature describe debilitating, sometime permanent, motor weakness and chronic neuropathic pain in young workers exposed to 1-BP as part of the spray adhesive used in foam cushion manufacturing. In one series of case reports of peripheral neuropathy associated with high level 1-BP use, affected employees had a 7-hour TWA exposure to 1-BP of 108 ppm [Majersik et al. 2007]. In a study of employees working in a 1-BP production facility, investigators found decreased vibration sense, decreased conduction velocity in sensory nerves, difficulty in digit recall, and decreased visual tracking ability [Ichihara et al. 2004]. This study found no motor deficits. Inhalational exposure studies on rats exposed to 200–

800 ppm 1-BP over several weeks revealed both motor and sensory neuropathies [Ichihara et al. 2000]. 1-BP has also been associated with adverse effects on the reproductive system [NIH 2003].

Human exposure to 1-BP can be assessed using a serum bromide level. This test is not usually available as a routine laboratory test. The results of a serum bromide level may not be available for several days, so this test is used to confirm an exposure, rather than to help establish an initial diagnosis. As per Goldfrank's Toxicological Emergencies, "Normal serum bromide concentrations are less than 500 mg/L" (this converts to 500 mcg/mL). Background levels of bromide result from intake of trace bromide in water due to absorption from surrounding rocks/soil containing bromide, produce treated with bromide-containing fumigants (methyl bromide and ethylene dibromide) and not washed thoroughly before eating, taking over-the-counter medications that contain bromide (e.g., dextromethorphan bromide used as a cough suppressant in cold medicine, brompheniramine maleate used as an antihistamine, bromo-seltzer, etc.), or after general anesthesia with halothane [Flomenbaum et al. 2006]. Toxicity from bromide had been reported with acute exposure to methyl bromide fumigant, overdose of medications containing bromide, or ingestion of bromide-containing neutralizers used in permanent wave hair products [Perez and McKay 2007]. Because the owner involved in the initial exposure incident did not have a serum bromide level done prior to this incident, we have no baseline for comparison to determine if the serum bromide level increased as a result of his exposure. However, the serum bromide level of 144 mcg/mL at the time of the exposure is well under the 1250 mcg/mL level associated with adverse health effects.

A laboratory finding of immediate use in determining exposure to 1-BP and other bromides is the chloride level on a routine standard metabolic assay. Depending on the equipment used to run the test, the chloride level may be elevated because of the bromide ion being counted as a chloride ion [Burkhart 2006]. Bromide can also be measured in the urine. This test was developed and evaluated against inhalational 1-BP exposure in workers exposed via use of spray adhesives; however, this test is not widely available [Hanley et al. 2006].

Full-shift sampling for 1-BP conducted at Facility 1 resulted in PBZ air concentrations of 40 ppm for the operator and 17 ppm for the cashier. This operator's exposure to 1-BP was well in excess of the current ACGIH TLV of 10 ppm. This operator ran a high number of loads on the day of sampling and cooked the solvent after each load, a practice that is not recommended by the manufacturer. Even the cashier, who did not operate the machine, had a PBZ air concentration that exceeded the recommended level, indicating that 1-BP poses a potential hazard to other employees in this facility (e.g., press operators who work next to the machines). Area air samples confirmed the release of high concentrations of 1-BP into

DISCUSSION
(CONTINUED)

the environment surrounding the machine. At this facility, air concentrations of 1-BP were higher in the morning, possibly because the general ventilation system was turned off during that time.

Partial shift sampling was conducted at the other three facilities because the owners requested that we remove the sampling equipment once they had finished running the dry cleaning machines. However, employees can have continued exposure to 1-BP after the last load is finished because of existing contamination in the environment. This exposure can be significant for facilities that do not have good general dilution ventilation or whose ventilation systems are not always in operation. PBZ concentrations ranging from 15 to 160 ppm were found in these 3.5- to 4-hour PBZ air samples collected at facilities 2, 3, and 4. The highest concentration (160 ppm) was measured at Facility 4. Although only one load was run by this operator, most of his time was spent cooking the solvent. Even if the operator had no further exposure to 1-BP during this work day, his full-shift PBZ concentration would be well in excess of the ACGIH TLV. An area air sample collected behind the machine at this facility confirmed the release of a high concentration of 1-BP into the work environment (170 ppm), again indicating a potential hazard to others in this work area. Machine leaks may have contributed to the high exposures; the owner had converted the machine himself and indicated that he had difficulty finding the correct materials for the conversion. Opening the front door of this facility and using an exhaust fan near the dry cleaning machine may have helped to keep this cashier's exposure low (2.4 ppm) on the day of sampling. This improvement was evident from the marked decrease in solvent odor after the fan was turned on and the front door was opened.

CONCLUSIONS

The NIOSH evaluation revealed that exposures to 1-BP can exceed the ACGIH TLV for 1-BP even for employees who do not operate the machines. It is expected that 1-BP exposures on a given day can be higher or lower at a given facility depending on work volume and work practices. Although we cannot make definitive conclusions based on our limited sampling, the highest concentrations of 1-BP were found at the two facilities that had converted the machines themselves and were cooking the solvent, a practice that had been performed widely for perc but is no longer recommended by the manufacturers for 1-BP operation. Further evaluation is needed to understand the relative contributions to the overall 1-BP exposures from possible machine leaks and practices such as cooking the solvent. This evaluation has shown that operators often rely on natural ventilation (opening doors and windows) for controlling exposures to 1-BP. This is not a good practice because weather conditions may preclude it. Although one owner reported transient symptoms consistent with general solvent exposure, we found no evidence of symptoms suggesting peripheral neuropathy in dry cleaners using 1-BP.

RECOMMENDATIONS

Based on our findings, we have several recommendations to create more healthful work places. We encourage owners of dry cleaning establishments to use these recommendations to develop an action plan based, if possible, on the hierarchy of controls approach (Appendix A: Occupational Exposure Limits and Health Effects). This approach groups actions by their likely effectiveness in reducing or removing hazards. In most cases, the preferred approach is to eliminate hazardous materials or processes and install engineering controls to reduce exposure or shield employees. Until such controls are in place, or if they are not effective or feasible, administrative measures and/or personal protective equipment may be needed. If operators or employees develop symptoms consistent with 1-BP exposure (such as lightheadedness, headache, or nausea), they should leave the area until the source of the exposure has been indentified and remediated. If symptoms do not resolve shortly after leaving the work area, or if the individuals develop extremity muscle weakness or sensory problems, they should seek immediate medical attention and notify their healthcare provider of the potential exposure to 1-BP.

Elimination and Substitution

Elimination or substitution of a toxic/hazardous process material is a highly effective means for reducing hazards. Incorporating this strategy into the design or development phase of a project, commonly referred to as "prevention through design," is most effective because it reduces the need for additional controls in the future.

1. Consider switching to wet cleaning methods. A wide variety of garments that are currently dry cleaned can be wet cleaned satisfactorily while controlling fabric deterioration and shrinkage [Gottlieb et al. 1997]. Wet cleaning has fewer health and safety concerns, as well as a reduced burden of environmental regulations [NIOSH 1997a]. Other alternatives include selecting a dry cleaning machine that uses petroleum-based solvents; these solvents are generally considered less toxic, although they are flammable and present a fire hazard [NIOSH 1997a].

Engineering Controls

Engineering controls reduce employee exposures by removing the hazard from the process or placing a barrier between the hazard and the employee. Engineering controls are very effective at protecting employees without placing primary responsibility of implementation on the employee.

1. Isolate machines from other work areas to reduce the exposure of employees who do not run the machine, such as press operators and cashiers.

2. Use LEV at or near the machine door to reduce worker exposure during machine loading and unloading and while performing maintenance. Airflow capacity through a retrofit hood should not be less than 100 times the door opening area in square feet (i.e., a 4 ft² door opening would need a flow rate of at least 400 cfm). The exhaust hood should be isolated from crossdrafts caused by general ventilation, floor or other shop fans, and high personnel traffic areas [NIOSH 1997b].

3. Use general ventilation to dilute background 1-BP concentrations. Generally accepted guidelines recommend 12 air changes per hour with a minimum of 30 cfm of outside air per person for dry cleaning establishments. The direction of airflow should move from a clean area (customer counters) to one that is less clean (dry cleaning machine area). A qualified ventilation system contractor should be contacted for assistance [NIOSH 1997b].

Administrative Controls

Administrative controls are management-dictated work practices and policies to reduce or prevent exposures to workplace hazards. The effectiveness of administrative changes in work practices for controlling workplace hazards is dependent on management commitment and employee acceptance. Regular monitoring and reinforcement are necessary to ensure that control policies and procedures are not circumvented in the name of convenience or production.

1. Use a qualified technician to convert the machines from perc to 1-BP to ensure the use of proper materials for replacement parts (e.g., gaskets), correct machine settings, and proper safety measures during the process.

2. Follow manufacturer guidelines on the use of ventilation, temperature, and system settings when using 1-BP.

3. Conduct air sampling periodically for 1-BP and whenever changes in work practices, procedures, or ventilation may affect employee exposures.

4. Do not cook the solvent. The manufacturer of Dry-Solv states that, unlike perc, the solvent does not require cooking.

5. Keep the machine door closed except when loading and unloading.

6. Advise the operator to keep his or her head out of the machine and stay as far away as possible from the door when loading and unloading. A tool with a long handle could be used to retrieve clothes from the back of the drum.

7. Use the full drying period, as cutting drying periods short may cause solvent to remain on the items and increase operator exposure.

8. Consider limiting the number of loads per day to reduce exposures below the OELs.

Personal Protective Equipment

PPE is the least effective means for controlling employee exposures. Proper use of PPE requires a comprehensive program, and calls for a high level of employee involvement and commitment to be effective. The use of PPE requires the choice of the appropriate equipment to reduce the hazard and the development of supporting programs such as training, change-out schedules, and medical assessment if needed. PPE should not be relied upon as the sole method for limiting employee exposures. Rather, PPE should be used until engineering and administrative controls can be demonstrated to be effective in limiting exposures to acceptable levels.

1. Wear safety glasses/goggles and gloves appropriate for 1-BP when handling the solvent as the Dry-Solv Material Safety Data Sheet suggests. Viton® or SilverShield® gloves offer the best protection.

2. Ensure that employees whose exposures can exceed the ACGIH TLV wear respirators until ventilation and administrative controls can be demonstrated to reduce employee exposures below applicable guidelines.

3. Instruct employees at Facility 1 to wear a minimum of an elastomeric half-mask air-purifying respirator with organic vapor cartridges, because air sample results indicate that the operator and cashier were exposed to 1-BP above the ACGIH TLV of 10 ppm. This respirator has an assigned protection factor of 10, meaning that exposures would be expected to be reduced by a factor of 10 if the respirator is properly fitted and worn in full accordance with the OSHA respirator standard. At Facility 4, the operator's exposure was much higher, indicating the need for a respirator with a higher assigned protection factor if cooking solvent is continued. This would include a minimum of a full facepiece air-purifying respirator or a powered air purifying respirator equipped with organic vapor cartridges. Although full-shift air sampling was not conducted at Facilities 2 or 3, it is possible that operators' full-shift exposures could exceed the 10 ppm guideline depending on the workload and other factors. We recommend conducting additional full-shift sampling at these facilities over multiple days to determine if respiratory protection is needed as an interim measure until additional ventilation and administrative controls are implemented.

RECOMMENDATIONS
(CONTINUED)

4. Ensure that all applicable requirements of the OSHA Respiratory Protection Standard (29 CFR 1910.134) are met where respirators are used. This includes medical screening, annual fit testing, training on the proper use and limitations of the respirator, and instruction on how to properly clean and store the respirator. A Small Entity Compliance Guide for the OSHA Respiratory Protection Standard is available at http://www.osha.gov/Publications/SECG_RPS/secg_rps.html. Additional information regarding respirator cartridge changeout is also available online at http://www.osha.gov/SLTC/etools/respiratory/change_schedule.html.

Other Recommendations

OSHA has a consultation service that is free to businesses that may prove helpful in conducting air sampling and establishing a respirator program. This service is separate from the OSHA compliance office, and use of its services cannot result in citations. Please see the OSHA website for further information at http://www.osha.gov/dcsp/smallbusiness/consult.html.

REFERENCES

American Drycleaner [2007]. Most drycleaners will consider alternatives. American Drycleaner 74(6):8.

Burkhart KK [2006]. Methyl bromide and other fumigants. In: Flomenbaum NE, Goldfrank LR, Hoffman RS, Howland MA, Lewin NA, Nelson LS eds. Goldfrank's toxicological emergencies. 8th ed. New York: McGraw-Hill Companies, Inc., pp. 1556–1563.

CDC (Centers for Disease Control and Prevention) [2008]. Neurologic illness associated with occupational exposure to the solvent 1-Bromopropane – New Jersey and Pennsylvania, 2007–2008. MMWR 57(48):1300–1302.

CFR. Code of Federal Regulations. Washington, DC: U.S. Government Printing Office, Office of the Federal Register.

Flomenbaum NE, Goldfrank LR, Hoffman RS, Howland MA, Lewin NA, Nelson LS, eds [2006]. Goldfrank's toxicological emergencies. 8th ed. New York: McGraw-Hill Companies, Inc. [http://elib.cdc.gov:2090/Document/Document.aspx?FxId=68&DocId=1&SessionId=1205F29GMKJWMRKL]. Date accessed: April 2010.

Gottlieb R, Goodheart J, Sinsheimer P, Tranby C, Bechtel L [1997]. Wet cleaning vs. dry cleaning of clothes. Research Note 97-14 from report "Evaluation and Demonstration of Wet Cleaning

Alternatives to Perchloroethylene-Based Garment Care." California Environmental Protection Agency Air Resources Board. December 1997. [http://www.arb.ca.gov/research/resnotes/notes/97-14.htm]. Date accessed: June 2010.

Hanley KW, Petersen M, Curwin BD, Sanderson WT [2006]. Urinary bromide and breathing zone concentrations of 1-bromopropane from workers exposed to flexible foam spray adhesives. Ann Occup Hyg 50(6):599–607.

Ichihara G, Kitoh J, Yu X, Asaeda N, Iwai H, Kumazawa T, Shibata E, Yamada T, Wang H, Xie Z, Takeuchi Y [2000]. 1-Bromopropane, an alternative to ozone layer depleting solvents, is dose-dependently neurotoxic to rats in long-term inhalation exposure. Toxicol Sci 55(1):116–123.

Majersik JJ, Caravati EM, Steffens JD [2007]. Severe neurotoxicity associated with exposure to the solvent 1-bromopropane (n-propyl bromide). Clin Toxicol 44(3):270–276.

McAneny DJ [2007]. N.J. forcing dry cleaners to clean up their act. New Jersey On-Line LLC [www.nj.com/south/index.ssf/2007/12/nj_forcing_dry_cleaners_to_cle.html]. Date accessed: June 2010.

NIH [2003]. NTP-CERHR monograph: The potential human reproductive and developmental effects of 1-bromopropane. Research Triangle Park, NC. U.S. Department of Health and Human Services, National Toxicology Program, Center for the Evaluation of Risks to Human Reproduction, NIH Publication No. 04-4479.

NIOSH [1997a]. Hazard Control HC17: Control to exposure of percholroethylene in commerical drycleaning (Substitution). U.S. Department of Health and Human Services, Centers for Disease Control and Prevention, National Institute for Occupational Safety and Health, DHHS (NIOSH) Publication 97-155 [http://www.cdc.gov/niosh/hc17.html]. Date accessed: June 2010.

NIOSH [1997b]. Hazard Control HC19: Control to exposure of percholroethylene in commerical drycleaning (Ventilation). U.S. Department of Health and Human Services, Centers for Disease Control and Prevention, National Institute for Occupational Safety and Health, DHHS (NIOSH) Publication 97-157 [http://www.cdc.gov/niosh/hc19.html]. Date accessed: June 2010.

NIOSH [2001]. Hazard evaluation and technical assistance report: Trilithic Inc., Indianapolis, IN. By Reh CM, Nemhauser JB. U.S. Department of Health and Human Services, Centers for Disease Control and Prevention, National Institute for Occupational Safety and Health, NIOSH HETA Report No. 2000-0233-2845.

NIOSH [2002]. Hazard evaluation and technical assistance report: STN Cushion Company, Cincinnati, OH. By Harney JM, Hess J, Reh CM, Trout D. U.S. Department of Health and Human Services, Centers for Disease Control and Prevention, National Institute for Occupational Safety and Health, NIOSH HETA Report No. 2000-0410-2891.

NIOSH [2003]. Hazard evaluation and technical assistance report: Marx Industries Inc., Thomasville, NC. By Harney JM, Nemhauser JB, Reh CM, Trout D. U.S. Department of Health and Human Services, Centers for Disease Control and Prevention, National Institute for Occupational Safety and Health, NIOSH HETA Report No. 1999-0260-2906.

NIOSH [2009]. NIOSH manual of analytical methods (NMAM®). 4th ed. Schlecht PC, O'Connor PF, eds. Cincinnati, OH: U.S. Department of Health and Human Services, Centers for Disease Control and Prevention, National Institute for Occupational Safety and Health, DHHS (NIOSH) Publication 94-113 (August 1994); 1st Supplement Publication 96-135, 2nd Supplement Publication 98-119; 3rd Supplement 2003-154. [http://www.cdc.gov/niosh/docs/2003-154/]. Date accessed: June 2010.

NJ DEP [2010a]. Notice of Rule Proposal – Control and Prohibition of Air Pollution by Toxic Substances; N.J A.C. 7:27-17. [http://www.state.nj.us/dep//rules/proposals/121707b.pdf]. Date accessed: June 2010.

NJ DEP [2010b]. Dry Cleaner Equipment Replacement Reimbursement Program. [http://www.state.nj.us/dep/enforcement/drycleanergrant.html]. Date accessed: June 2010.

Perez A, McKay C [2007]. Halogens (bromine, iodine and chlorine compounds) In: Shannon MW, Borron SW, Burns MJ, eds. Haddad and Winchester's clinical management of poisoning and drug overdose. 4th ed. Philadelphia: Elsevier Inc., pp. 1385–1397.

Appendix A: Occupational Exposure Limits and Health Effects

In evaluating the hazards posed by workplace exposures, NIOSH investigators use both mandatory (legally enforceable) and recommended OELs for chemical, physical, and biological agents as a guide for making recommendations. OELs have been developed by Federal agencies and safety and health organizations to prevent the occurrence of adverse health effects from workplace exposures. Generally, OELs suggest levels of exposure that most employees may be exposed up to 10 hours per day, 40 hours per week for a working lifetime without experiencing adverse health effects. However, not all employees will be protected from adverse health effects even if their exposures are maintained below these levels. A small percentage may experience adverse health effects because of individual susceptibility, a preexisting medical condition, and/or hypersensitivity (allergy). In addition, some hazardous substances may act in combination with other workplace exposures, the general environment, or with medications or personal habits of the employee to produce health effects even if the occupational exposures are controlled at the level set by the exposure limit. Also, some substances can be absorbed by direct contact with the skin and mucous membranes in addition to being inhaled, which contributes to the individual's overall exposure.

Most OELs are expressed as a TWA exposure. A TWA refers to the average exposure during a normal 8- to 10-hour workday. Some chemical substances and physical agents have recommended STEL or ceiling values where health effects are caused by exposures over a short period. Unless otherwise noted, the STEL is a 15-minute TWA exposure that should not be exceeded at any time during a workday, and the ceiling limit is an exposure that should not be exceeded at any time.

In the United States, OELs have been established by federal agencies, professional organizations, state and local governments, and other entities. Some OELs are legally enforceable limits, while others are recommendations. The U.S. Department of Labor OSHA PELs (29 CFR 1910 [general industry]; 29 CFR 1926 [construction industry]; and 29 CFR 1917 [maritime industry]) are legal limits enforceable in workplaces covered under the Occupational Safety and Health Act. NIOSH RELs are recommendations based on a critical review of the scientific and technical information available on a given hazard and the adequacy of methods to identify and control the hazard. NIOSH RELs can be found in the *NIOSH Pocket Guide to Chemical Hazards* [NIOSH 2005]. NIOSH also recommends different types of risk management practices (e.g., engineering controls, safe work practices, employee education/training, personal protective equipment, and exposure and medical monitoring) to minimize the risk of exposure and adverse health effects from these hazards. Other OELs that are commonly used and cited in the United States include the TLVs recommended by ACGIH, a professional organization, and the WEELs recommended by the American Industrial Hygiene Association, another professional organization. The TLVs and WEELs are developed by committee members of these associations from a review of the published, peer-reviewed literature. They are not consensus standards. ACGIH TLVs are considered voluntary exposure guidelines for use by industrial hygienists and others trained in this discipline "to assist in the control of health hazards" [ACGIH 2009]. WEELs have been established for some chemicals "when no other legal or authoritative limits exist" [AIHA 2009].

Outside the United States, OELs have been established by various agencies and organizations and include both legal and recommended limits. Since 2006, the Berufsgenossenschaftliches Institut für Arbeitsschutz (German Institute for Occupational Safety and Health) has maintained a database of international OELs from European Union member states, Canada (Québec), Japan, Switzerland, and the United States available at http://www.dguv.de/bgia/en/gestis/limit_values/index.jsp. The database contains international limits for over 1250 hazardous substances and is updated annually.

Employers should understand that not all hazardous chemicals have specific OSHA PELs, and for some agents the legally enforceable and recommended limits may not reflect current health-based information.

However, an employer is still required by OSHA to protect its employees from hazards even in the absence of a specific OSHA PEL. OSHA requires an employer to furnish employees a place of employment free from recognized hazards that cause or are likely to cause death or serious physical harm [Occupational Safety and Health Act of 1970 (Public Law 91–596, sec. 5(a)(1))]. Thus, NIOSH investigators encourage employers to make use of other OELs when making risk assessment and risk management decisions to best protect the health of their employees. NIOSH investigators also encourage the use of the traditional hierarchy of controls approach to eliminate or minimize identified workplace hazards. This includes, in order of preference, the use of: (1) substitution or elimination of the hazardous agent, (2) engineering controls (e.g , local exhaust ventilation, process enclosure, dilution ventilation), (3) administrative controls (e.g., limiting time of exposure, employee training, work practice changes, medical surveillance), and (4) personal protective equipment (e.g., respiratory protection, gloves, eye protection, hearing protection). Control banding, a qualitative risk assessment and risk management tool, is a complementary approach to protecting employee health that focuses resources on exposure controls by describing how a risk needs to be managed. Information on control banding is available at http://www.cdc.gov/niosh/topics/ ctrlbanding/. This approach can be applied in situations where OELs have not been established or can be used to supplement the OELs, when available.

1-Bromopropane

As with other solvents, occupational exposure to 1-BP may occur via both inhalation and skin absorption. Health effects related to overexposure to 1-BP (and many other solvents) may include irritation of the eyes, mucous membranes, upper respiratory tract, and skin. At higher levels of exposure, central nervous system depression (characterized by headache and dizziness, and possibly loss of consciousness) may occur.

Neither NIOSH nor OSHA has OELs for 1-BP. However, NIOSH is developing an REL. The ACGIH has set a TLV of 10 ppm for 1-BP as an 8-hour TWA exposure [ACGIH 2009]. The primary basis for the TLV is liver damage, embryo/fetal damage, and neurotoxicity.

The U.S. EPA determined that 1-BP is acceptable for use as a substitute for ozone-depleting substances in metal cleaning, electronics cleaning, and precision cleaning applications. This determination was based upon the conclusion that 1-BP exposures in the range of 17–30 ppm in such applications would not likely cause adverse human reproductive effects. However, the U.S. EPA also proposed that the use of 1-BP in aerosol or adhesive applications is not acceptable based on higher than anticipated workplace exposures. U.S. EPA does not regulate the use of solvents in dry cleaning under the Significant New Alternatives Policy Program [72 Fed. Reg. 30142(2007)].

Previous investigations have linked peripheral neuropathy to high level 1-BP exposure in electronics degreasing [NIOSH 2001] and foam cushion manufacturing [NIOSH 2002; NIOSH 2003]. Case reports in the medical literature describe debilitating, sometimes permanent, motor weakness and chronic neuropathic pain in young workers exposed to 1-BP as part of the spray adhesive used in foam cushion manufacturing. In one series of case reports of peripheral neuropathy associated with high level 1-BP use, affected employees had 7-hour TWA exposure to 1-BP of 108 ppm [Majersik et al. 2007]. In a study of employees working in a 1-BP production facility, investigators found decreased vibration sense, decreased conduction velocity in sensory nerves, difficulty in digit recall, and decreased visual tracking ability [Ichihara et al. 2004]. This study found no motor deficits. Inhalational exposure studies done on rats exposed to 200–800 ppm 1-BP over several weeks revealed both motor and sensory neuropathies [Ichihara et al. 2000].

Human exposure to 1-BP can be assessed using a serum bromide level. This test is not usually available as a routine laboratory test. The results of a serum bromide level may not be available for several days, so this test is used to confirm an exposure, rather than to help establish an initial diagnosis. However, a laboratory finding of immediate use in determining exposure to 1-BP and other bromides is the chloride level on a routine standard metabolic assay. Depending on the equipment used to run the test, the chloride level may be elevated because of the bromide ion being counted as a chloride ion [Burkhart 2006]. Bromide can also be measured in the urine. This test was developed and evaluated against inhalational 1-BP exposure in workers exposed via use of spray adhesives; however, this test is not widely available [Hanley et al. 2006].

References

ACGIH [2009]. 2009 TLVs® and BEIs®: threshold limit values for chemical substances and physical agents and biological exposure indices. Cincinnati, OH: American Conference of Governmental Industrial Hygienists.

AIHA [2009]. AIHA 2009 Emergency response planning guidelines (ERPG) & workplace environmental exposure levels (WEEL) handbook. Fairfax, VA: American Industrial Hygiene Association.

Burkhart KK [2006] Methyl bromide and other fumigants. In: Flomenbaum NE, Goldfrank LR, Hoffman RS, Howland MA, Lewin NA, Nelson LS eds. Goldfrank's toxicological emergencies. 8th ed. New York: McGraw-Hill Companies, Inc., pp. 1556–1563.

CFR. Code of Federal Regulations. Washington, DC: U.S. Government Printing Office, Office of the Federal Register.

72 Fed. Reg. 30142 [2007]. Protection of stratospheric ozone: listing of substitutes for ozone-depleting substances-n-propyl bromide in solvent cleaning. (To be codified at 40 CFR Part 82) [http://www.epa.gov/fedrgstr/EPA-AIR/2007/May/Day-30/a9707.pdf]. Date accessed: June 2010.

Hanley KW, Petersen M, Curwin BD, Sanderson WT [2006]. Urinary bromide and breathing zone concentrations of 1-bromopropane from workers exposed to flexible foam spray adhesives. Ann Occup Hyg 50(6):599–607.

Ichihara G, Kitoh J, Yu X, Asaeda N, Iwai H, Kumazawa T, Shibata E, Yamada T, Wang H, Xie Z, Takeuchi Y [2000]. 1-Bromopropane, an alternative to ozone layer depleting solvents, is dose-dependently neurotoxic to rats in long-term inhalation exposure. Toxicol Sci 55(1):116–123.

Ichihara G, Li W, Shibata E, Ding X, Wang H, Liang Y, Peng S, Itohara S, Kamijima M, Fan Q, Zhang Y, Zhong E, Wu X, Valentine WM, Takeuchi Y [2004]. Neurologic abnormalities in workers of a 1-bromopropane factory. Environ Health Perspect 112(13):1319–1325.

Majersik JJ, Caravati EM, Steffens JD [2007]. Severe neurotoxicity associated with exposure to the solvent 1-bromopropane (n-propyl bromide). Clin Toxicol 44(3):270–276.

NIOSH [2001]. Hazard evaluation and technical assistance report: Trilithic Inc., Indianapolis, IN. By Reh CM, Nemhauser JB. U.S. Department of Health and Human Services, Centers for Disease Control and Prevention, National Institute for Occupational Safety and Health, NIOSH HETA Report No. 2000-0233-2845.

NIOSH [2002]. Hazard evaluation and technical assistance report: STN Cushion Company, Cincinnati, OH. By Harney JM, Hess J, Reh CM, Trout D. U.S. Department of Health and Human Services, Centers for Disease Control and Prevention, National Institute for Occupational Safety and Health, NIOSH HETA Report No. 2000-0410-2891.

NIOSH [2003]. Hazard evaluation and technical assistance report: Marx Industries Inc., Thomasville, NC. By Harney JM, Nemhauser JB, Reh CM, Trout D. U.S. Department of Health and Human Services,

Centers for Disease Control and Prevention, National Institute for Occupational Safety and Health, NIOSH HETA Report No. 1999-0260-2906.

NIOSH [2005]. NIOSH pocket guide to chemical hazards. Cincinnati, OH: U.S. Department of Health and Human Services, Centers for Disease Control and Prevention, National Institute for Occupational Safety and Health, DHHS (NIOSH) Publication No. 2005-149. [http://www.cdc.gov/niosh/npg/]. Date accessed: June 2010.

ACKNOWLEDGMENTS AND AVAILABILITY OF REPORT

The Hazard Evaluations and Technical Assistance Branch (HETAB) of the National Institute for Occupational Safety and Health (NIOSH) conducts field investigations of possible health hazards in the workplace. These investigations are conducted under the authority of Section 20(a)(6) of the Occupational Safety and Health Act of 1970, 29 U.S.C. 669(a)(6) which authorizes the Secretary of Health and Human Services, following a written request from any employers or authorized representative of employees, to determine whether any substance normally found in the place of employment has potentially toxic effects in such concentrations as used or found. HETAB also provides, upon request, technical and consultative assistance to federal, state, and local agencies; labor; industry; and other groups or individuals to control occupational health hazards and to prevent related trauma and disease.

The findings and conclusions in this report are those of the authors and do not necessarily represent the views of NIOSH. Mention of any company or product does not constitute endorsement by NIOSH. In addition, citations to websites external to NIOSH do not constitute NIOSH endorsement of the sponsoring organizations or their programs or products. Furthermore, NIOSH is not responsible for the content of these websites. All Web addresses referenced in this document were accessible as of the publication date.

This report was prepared by Judith Eisenberg and Jessica Ramsey of HETAB, Division of Surveillance, Hazard Evaluations and Field Studies. Health communication assistance was provided by Stefanie Evans. Editorial assistance was provided by Ellen Galloway. Desktop publishing was performed by Robin Smith.

Copies of this report have been sent to the New Jersey Department of Health and Senior Services and the Occupational Safety and Health Administration Regional Office. This report is not copyrighted and may be freely reproduced. The report may be viewed and printed at www.cdc.gov/niosh/hhe. Copies may be purchased from the National Technical Information Service at 5825 Port Royal Road, Springfield, Virginia 22161.

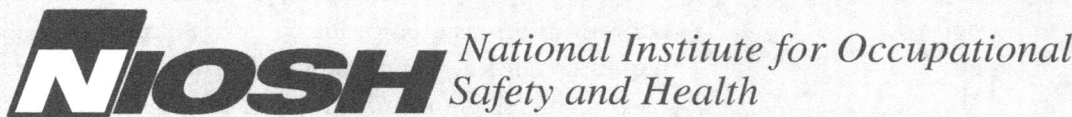

National Institute for Occupational Safety and Health

Delivering on the Nation's promise: Safety and health at work for all people through research and prevention.

To receive NIOSH documents or information about occupational safety and health topics, contact NIOSH at:

1-800-CDC-INFO (1-800-232-4636)

TTY: 1-888-232-6348

E-mail: cdcinfo@cdc.gov

or visit the NIOSH web site at: **www.cdc.gov/niosh.**

For a monthly update on news at NIOSH, subscribe to NIOSH eNews by visiting **www.cdc.gov/niosh/eNews.**

SAFER • HEALTHIER • PEOPLE™

www.ingramcontent.com/pod-product-compliance
Lightning Source LLC
Chambersburg PA
CBHW080941290526
45795CB00007BA/2849